VOICE

LIFE

Living The Abundant Life
Beyond 3 Score And 10

Eunice Downing-Jackson

VOICE LIFE

Voice Life
Living The Abundant Life Beyond 3 Score And 10
By: Eunice Downing-Jackson

Published By: Eunice 4 A Healthier You
Email: Eunice4AHealthierYou@gmail.com

Voice Life
Website/Blog : Voicelife120.com
Email: Voicelife120@gmail.com

Unless otherwise noted, scriptures are quoted from:
King James Version, and New King James Version

Proofreader: Rose Marie Haughton

ISBN-13:978-1-7325828-0-4 (Paperback)

DEDICATION

To my husband Truly H. Jackson, daughter Chimeka Crawford
and my West Angeles Church of God In Christ Family.

❖

Say it!

Voice life... Say it!

I can do all things through Christ who strengthens me. Say it.

He fills my mouth with good things. Say it.

He renews my youth as the young eagles. Say it.

Say it, believe it, receive it, and live it.

Poem written By Clara U. Downing

Author of: Hush, Mother Is Praying: Her Life Is A Testimony, and Living in the Secret Place.

Foreword

As children of God, we can contribute to the body of Christ at every stage of our life. Eunice Downing-Jackson wrote a compelling book which challenges us to take control and be proactive when it comes to managing our health, loving life and focusing on your purpose.

Voice Life, gives a personal and researched account of lifestyles as you transition into senior status and beyond. It is inspirational and provides educational tips for living a longer, more vibrant life, as well as encouraging others. Helpful resources are in the back of the book for tracking results.

Lady Mae L. Blake,
First Lady, West Angeles Church of God in Christ,
Author of several books including, Class Act 1 and Class Act 2, Gems from Lady Mae, and Getting Rid of the "Stuff" that Clutters your life.

About The Author

Eunice Downing-Jackson likes to think of herself as an undercover agent for God, she is either on an assignment or preparing for an assignment. She prefers to let her actions and contributions define her. God has given her the gift of encouragement to edify the body of Christ.

Eunice is an active member of West Angeles Church of God in Christ for more than 35 years, where she continues to be blessed by the teaching and the anointing of Bishop Charles E. Blake and Lady Mae L. Blake.

She also worked in corporate America for more than 35 years in the insurance industry underwriting risk. She received one of her favorite assignments from God during planning stages of the Cathedral. She shared the dream with Bishop Blake in a letter. Bishop Blake called while she was at work and said, "I know you will be involved in some way, but at this time I don't know how".

Eunice felt her way of getting involved was to participate in the building fund campaign. However, about ten years later, while working as an employee for a different insurance carrier, she returned from her lunch break, to find a builder's risk submission on her desk for the West Angeles Church, it was for the Cathedral. She was surprised! Not only was she given permission to work on the account by her employer, the insurance broker allowed her to select what she felt was the best coverage and premium. This is a demonstration of God's favor and how He will position you to be of service to others. Eunice felt this was an assignment from God.

Voice Life is another assignment from God. Eunice's desire to create a healthier lifestyle for her family, led her on an unexpected journey where health and wellness became part of her ministry. She feels an obligation to encourage people to take control of their health and well being, by living life and growing gracefully under the power of the Holy Spirit focusing on an abundant life beyond 3 score and 10.

Eunice along with her husband Truly Hicks Jackson lives in Los Angeles, Ca.

Acknowledgements

Special thanks to Jehovah God, my provider, who inspired me through the precious Holy Spirit to share this message. I would also like to acknowledge:

Bishop Charles E. Blake and Lady Mae L. Blake of West Angeles Church of God In Christ, thank you for your leadership and being a positive role model. I wish you a long, healthy, vibrant life, that is full of joy.

Rev. Elijah Starr, retired Associate Pastor, Sunday school teacher and prayer warrior for his consultation and prayers.

My sister Rose Haughton for consultation, editorial work in the preparation of the manuscript and keeping me focused.

Janice Smallwood-McKenzie, Networking Coach and Author for her encouragement.

Shirley J. Patterson, Certified Performance Coach who continues to support me in my journey.

Yvonne Gipson-Johnson, Prayer Ministry Director of West Angeles C.O.G.I.C, who continues to speak the ministry of health into my life.

Two special friends, Linda Brimberry and Joan Reeves who have been with me through thick and thin, who always seem to have the right words at the right time.

My mother and family who I love, they keep me inspired and grounded.

My loving husband, Truly Jackson and daughter Chimeka Crawford for their love, support and encouragement!!

Introduction

My grandmother always said "read the bible for yourself and if you can only make it to one service, make sure it is Sunday school. Sunday school is where you study the word, ask questions and discuss what you have heard and learned." I was impressed with her knowledge of the Bible and the way she compared it to modern times.

I have asked myself why am I writing this book? I am not a scientist, nor a medical doctor, but a Blessed Child of God. I have always felt that I had a book in me, but why *living beyond 80 years old?* I do know while writing this book, the research has answered so many of my questions regarding pre-flood and post-flood conditions and lifespan.

As I prayed, I knew God wanted me to write a book that would make a difference in the lives of others and give people hope. As I studied more and more about health and shared with various people that God sent across my path I had a desire to SCREAM "PEOPLE YOU NEED TO VOICE AND THINK LIFE NOT DEATH". Why? Because most of the people that I spoke to did not expect to see 90 years old; nor did they want to live to see 100. To be honest, I would probably say the same thing, if I felt my life was not productive. We cannot get weary in well doing… (Gal 6:9). When you have a relationship with God, you can affect positive change at any stage of your life. It is never too late and you are not alone.

VOICE LIFE

Table of Contents

VOICE LIFE

Chapter 1
Standing on The Word

I remember seeing my sister lying on the hospital bed on life support. It was in February of 2012. She was heavily sedated, hooked up to several IV fluid bags, on a breathing apparatus and other machines monitoring her vital signs of life. To my knowledge, my sister was not aware my father and I were present in the room with her.

As my father and I sat in the room watching over my sister, praying and quietly talking to each other, I could see and feel his deep concern. My father was a "rolling stone" with over 22 children. He was mumbling and kept saying this is my fourth born. He was probably thinking about the year before when he attended the funeral of his third born.

The doctor walked into my sister's hospital room with a cordial greeting to my father and I. The doctor engaged us in a casual conversation and shared how long he has been my sister's doctor and made comments about her well-known voicetress attitude.

The doctor began explaining to us the purpose of the equipment in the room. He explained the breathing machine was doing most of the work, as he pointed to the breathing monitors, I believe he stated my sister was breathing at 25% on her own. He pointed to the IV bags filled with fluids of various colors. He stated, whenever you see IV bags of many colors hooked up to a patient, it is not a good sign. He referred to the IV bags as Christmas lights which meant my sister had a poor immune system. When he finished his assessment, he told us that at most, my sister had two days to live.

The doctor did an amazing job of painting a vision of no hope and death for my sister. At the time, my father was the medical care decision maker for my sister. It seemed like the doctor assumed my father's decision would be to "pull the plug"; meaning take her off life support. My heart was grieving, I did not know what to do, and God knows I was happy I did not have to make the final decision. I never saw my father, who was 83 years old, as a Christian man. I was surprised, to hear my father sharing from his heart the word of God with the doctor. This was the first time my father was recognized as the primary decision maker of one of his children. He lost a son almost 19 years earlier who was 36 years old and often said there was nothing he could do. Maybe he felt God was giving him a second chance.

Suddenly, my father stopped talking. There was a pause. Then he said, "I cannot have her taken off life support because the bible says we are promised three score and ten and she is not 70 yet". The doctor came across as very negative and continued to paint the picture of no hope for my sister's recovery. I finally said to the doctor "we are a family that believe in miracles". My father continued to repeat "three score and ten" during the time the doctor was in the room and after the doctor left the room. Then my father said to me, " if they will give her some beans and goat's milk she will get better". He was serious.

My father stayed overnight at the hospital, in Ridgecrest, Ca; a small community located 150 miles outside of Los

Angeles, Ca. At first, I did not feel comfortable returning to Los Angeles and leaving him in Ridgecrest because of his health challenges, but he insisted. I thought to myself, what can happen; he is in a hospital.

My father sat in my sister's hospital room in a chair by her bed, praying through the night. I arrived the next day to see the medical staff rushing around. My father was pacing the floor in front of my sister's room. I was informed my sister had a "Code Blue". Once again the doctor, offered no hope of my sister surviving. He explained my sister's condition, and the effects of the resuscitation process which included broken ribs from the pressure of trying to revive her. My sister survived the "Code Blue" and there were no broken ribs. I felt this was a sign from God that she was going to recover; however, the doctor was not convinced. My father continued repeating three score and ten. You may find this difficult to believe, but the doctor was visibly upset.

Two days later, my sister was still alive, but her health continued to deteriorate. Around the third day, my father overheard the doctor giving the nurse instructions not to waste their resources on my sister, because she was not expected to live. My father really got upset; I had to calm him down. He actually said he wanted to jump on the doctor. The doctor later shared with me, they had to send a police patrol car to Bakersfield, Ca, which he said was about two hours away, to get blood for my sister. My father asked, if he was trying to say his daughter was not worth it. The doctor did not respond, instead he went through the stages leading up to death.

My sister developed another health issue, kidney problems and needed to be put on a dialysis machine. The hospital no longer had the equipment available for her health challenges. Not having an available kidney dialysis machine was a blessing, because my sister was transferred to a larger hospital in Lancaster, Ca. The Lancaster hospital staff had a positive attitude and spoke life not death. The staff encouraged the family to believe my sister would recover and said they are praying with us. My prayer warrior sister also arrived and stayed with my sister at the hospital in Lancaster.

After a week of prayer, my sister recovered and woke up. I told her, "thank God daddy was the decision maker because her primary doctor sounded pretty convincing to me." While I was visiting my sister, I notice her meal was beans and regular milk. God has a sense of humor. I guess the goat milk was not readily available. My sister recovered and went back to Ridgecrest, Ca Out of curiosity, I asked my sister, if she saw her primary doctor and what did he say? She said, she saw him walking in the hallway during a follow-up appointment with another doctor. She said he looked at her like he saw a ghost and said I thought you died; it is a miracle. She later found out that he requested to be released as her doctor.

Chapter 2
What is Old Age

I have heard three score and ten quoted so many times over the past years and accepted it as the average age for longevity. In talking to family, friends and associates over the years, most people start thinking they are nearing death when they are around their mid-seventies and eighties. Insurance life-expectancy tables stop once you are around 85 years old. To hear someone say, your parents or grandparents do not have a life expectancy, yet you see and talk to them every day can be emotional.

What is the definition of old? One definition is that you are considered old when you become eligible for Social Security benefits at age 65. According to the Webster New World College Dictionary, it is defined as advanced years of life, special human life, and when strength and vigor decline.

Webster's definition sounds reasonable to me because to some extent you have control over the aging process. You have a chronological or actual age which is based on when you were born and an effective or biological age which is based on your lifestyle. The NCBI published a research article: *"How old are you, really? Communicating chronic risk through 'effective age' of your body and organs"*. The research explores conditions under which years to your effective age are lost or gained with reference to various organs such as heart age, lung age due to behavioral exposures and certain risk factors. Under reasonable assumptions, the risks associated with specific behaviors can be expressed in terms of years gained or lost off your effective age.

Healthcare professionals and insurance companies make major decisions regarding your health, the type of treatment received, medical coverage and premiums based on key factors which include your age. I remember the first time I shared with my doctor that I was experiencing muscle and joint pain in my legs and feet when waking up in the mornings. The first thing that came out of his mouth was, "let's face it, you are getting old". At the time, I was in my late 40s, but who wants to hear "you are getting old." For the next several years, I assumed the change my body was going through was due to me getting older. I am sure my doctor's remarks accelerated my aging process.

Doctors probably say "you are getting old", because they do not know the reason for your health challenge and in some cases it sounds like a logical explanation. When you have a relationship with God, He will tell you what your body is lacking and point you in the right direction. Will you follow His direction? How many warnings will He have to give you? What will it take for you to take action? For me it was eating more fruits and vegetables and eating healthier. I was a meat and potatoes person and vegetables were seldom on my plate. Other than enjoying the taste of food and satisfying my hunger pains, I did not know the value of food as it related to health. If at all possible, I avoided being around people that I thought had colds or the flu. I felt getting one seasonal cold a year was normal. Although I occasionally got the flu, I personally felt my immune system was strong.

While in my early 40's God started putting people in my path who spoke about the benefits of eating colorful and a variety of fruits and vegetables. I heard what they were saying; however at the time, I still could not comprehend the benefits of eating more fruits and vegetables. On a weekly basis, I would alternate between apples, oranges, peaches and of course, I can't forget the bananas for my Frosted Flakes and Cheerios. For me, vegetables was for special occasions!

Over 10 years later, my daughter was enjoying the life of a college student, on the track and field team, and called home as needed. I always had a challenge getting her to take vitamins. I was surprised when she called inquiring about a company that sold encapsulated fruits and vegetables.   At the time it was 17 serving of fruits and vegetables in a juiced powder form. I was excited and ordered the product for the whole family.

Months later I realized, I was no longer experiencing pain when I woke up in the morning, which my doctor said was a result of getting old. The overall health results for my family were amazing. I am still thanking God, because this one simple change made a huge difference in my family's health and we now enjoy eating a variety fruits and vegetables. My body now craves fruits, vegetables including big salads and I eat very little meat.

It took me over 10 years to follow God's direction about eating healthier. It is a learning curve and I am still on the journey for a healthier lifestyle. I now visualize healthy foods and a rainbow of colors flowing through feeding my body and various organs good nutrition; omega 3s improving my brain; water hydrating my body, cushioning my bones and along with fiber pushing out impurities; and exercise helping my body to make it's own medicine.

I realized the impact of treatment as it related to age in 2007. At that time, I was 57 years old and was involved in a car accident. I fractured the upper part of my leg; I think it was called the tibia. I was asked to complete a medical questionnaire at the doctor's office. In completing the questionnaire, I realized the questions were geared towards determining my activity level, for example how often you exercise, the type of exercises, level of intensity and etc. The information is then used by the doctor and the insurance company to determine the level of treatment I would receive. A similar process is used to determine the value of a vehicle at the time of an accident, such as the age of your vehicle and how many miles on your vehicle. However, your body is not a vehicle, which can be replaced.

As I completed the questionnaire, I checked the highest level of activity for each category. I shared verbally with the orthopedic doctor that I was very active and recently purchased two new pairs of 3-inch high-heels which I expected to wear after my recovery without missing a

step or limping. The doctor had a puzzled looked on his face. I got the feeling he was thinking, you should be thankful to be alive. Yes, I was thankful and praising God for being alive. However, insurance companies may deny or limit certain coverage to reduce expenses. For example, originally the insurance company only allowed for a certain number of weeks for my therapy treatment. The orthopedic doctor and my primary doctor submitted a petition to the insurance company, on my behalf, for a time extension.

I could have replaced my vehicle which was totaled, with another vehicle within weeks of the accident. However, during the treatment and recovery process, God showed me the benefits of taking public transportation. I initially struggled mentally and physically through pain and frustration as I walked two to three blocks to the buses, up and down the stairs to and from the train stations. I was concerned that someone might knock me over because I was not moving fast enough or in their way, so I tried avoiding crowds. Before I knew it, I found myself walking better and faster, I started outrunning commuters half my age and younger. Of course, they were not aware we were racing. Winning boosted my confidence, my recovery time was quicker than expected and my body was in better condition than it was prior to the accident.

What is old age? It really is just a number. Focus on your health, mental attitude and your relationship with God!

VOICE LIFE

Chapter 3
Voice Life not Death

While talking to a colleague about healthy lifestyles, she referenced a book, and said, "you know, we were meant to live to 150, however, pollution and stress has affected our lifespan". I sarcastically thought to myself, 150 years? Quickly my mind started thinking, "the Bible says 3 score and 10, not sure what she is referring to, not sure about her Christian beliefs, she does refer to the Universe instead of God, she may be a little off with her thinking. I have no desire to get into a discussion with her about living 150 years".

God has a way of getting our attention. Several months later, while turning the pages of my Bible, I noticed a graph (figure 1, on the next page) in the Church of God in Christ Spirit Filled Bible, page 13, Ages of the Patriarchs (5:5). I cannot tell you how many times I have seen and read this graph. This time, it was an "aha" moment for me. Although I did not see 150 years, what I noticed was the comment about pollution having an effect which resulted in a shorter lifespan and I thought about the one-sided discussion with my colleague.

Prior to the flood, mankind's average life span was 900 years; however God was not happy with the sinful and evil acts of man along with their disobedience. God's heart was grieved, and He cursed man by

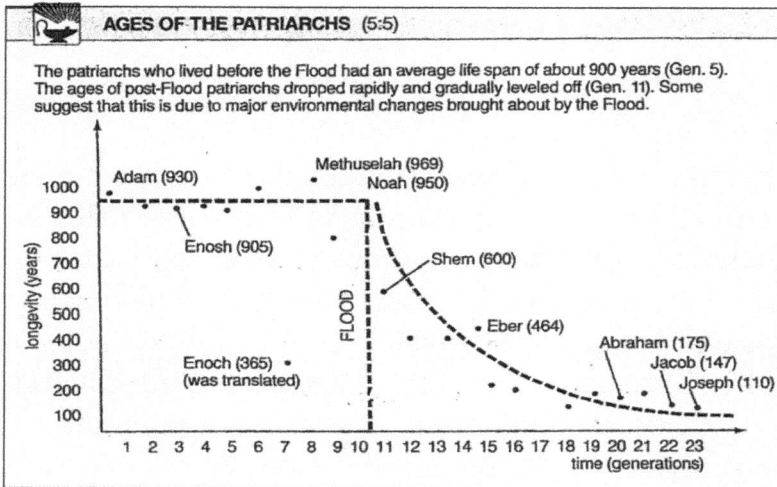

AGES OF THE PATRIARCHS (5:5)

The patriarchs who lived before the Flood had an average life span of about 900 years (Gen. 5). The ages of post-Flood patriarchs dropped rapidly and gradually leveled off (Gen. 11). Some suggest that this is due to major environmental changes brought about by the Flood.

Figure 1: Ages of the Patriarchs

limiting their days to 120 years. Genesis 6:3 - And *the Lord said, "My Spirit shall not strive with man forever, for he is indeed flesh; yet his days shall be one hundred and twenty years." (KJV)*

There are various opinions regarding the 120 years, some Bible scholars have expressed the following: It has nothing to do with man's life expectancy but with mercy. God is giving man 120 years to repent because the flood happened 120 years later. The flood was God way of cleansing the world of evil and disobedience.

Why do 120 years have to refer to the shortening of man's longevity or time period for repentance because of corruption? We can see from history, that both actually happened. God reducing the age expectancy to 120 years is not in conflict with Psalm 90:10 - *The days of our years are threescore years and ten; and if by reason of strength they be fourscore years, yet is their strength labour and sorrow; for it is soon cut off, and we fly away. (KJV)*

Moses wrote the book of Genesis and Psalm 90. Psalm 90 is referred to as "A Prayer of Moses the Man of God". In the prayer, Moses expresses thankfulness, and gives honor to God. He asked for mercy and forgiveness for the people of Israel. With the exception of the Israelites' little children who would be victims, Caleb son of Jephunneh and Joshua son of Nun, the Israelites were sentenced to 40 years in the wilderness because of their unbelief, complaining and rebellion, by God. (Numbers 14).

Numbers 14:26-35: *The Lord said to Moses and Aaron "How long will this wicked community grumble against me? I have heard the complaints of these grumbling Israelites. So tell them, 'As surely as I live, declares the Lord, I will do to you the very thing I heard you say: In this wilderness your bodies will fall—every one of you twenty years old or more who was counted in the census and who has grumbled against me. Not one of you will enter the land I swore with uplifted hand to make your home, except Caleb son of Jephunneh and Joshua son of Nun. As for your children that you said would be taken as plunder, I will bring them in to enjoy the land you have rejected. But as for you, your bodies will fall in this wilderness. Your children will be shepherds here for forty years, suffering for your unfaithfulness, until the last of your bodies lies in the wilderness. For forty years—one year for each of the forty days you explored the land—you will suffer for your sins and know what it is like to have me against you.' I, the Lord, have spoken, and I will surely do these things to this whole wicked community, which has banded together against me. They will meet their end in this wilderness; here they will die."* (NIV)

According to Matthew Henry Commentary on the Whole Bible, Moses taught the people of Israel to pray, and put words into their mouths which they might make use of in praying for repentance to the Lord. Psalm 90 may have been a daily prayer, which the Israelites said in their tents or said by the priests during tabernacle-service.

Psalm 90:10 is directed towards the Israelites. I was unable to find any documentation as to why Moses selected 70-80 as life expectancy. We do know because of God's death sentence, many of the Israelites were dying before they were 60 years old. After 40 years of wandering in the wilderness, the average life expectancy was probably 40-50. Is it possible the Israelites did not see themselves living any longer than 45?

As an intercessor, Psalm 90 was written by Moses to give Israelites hope in living beyond the average of 40 – 50 years? To voice and think life, not death? Proverbs 18:21 *Death and life are in the power of the tongue: and they that love it shall eat the fruit thereof (KJV).* Moses was 120 years old when he died.

Chapter 4
Take The Limits Off Life Expectancy

I started having discussions with family, friends, and strangers about the average life expectancy. Like myself, most of them said 80 and quoted 3 score and 10. A few reminded me that the 120 years in Genesis 6:3 is a curse which could be the reason why it is not referenced as much as 3 score and 10. However, when comparing 120 years to 70-80 years, 120 years is a blessing in modern-day times. No one I spoke to thought about living to 120 years as a blessing and got excited! It was difficult for them to visualize themselves living to 100 years old. I may feel the same way in a few years, that is why I enjoy listening to active, vibrant, healthy, positive "older" seniors and centenarians who are fulfilling God's purpose for their life.

A friend of mine who is a minister and Sunday school teacher in his 80s pointed out, Genesis 6:3 does not eliminate the pain and suffering you feel as you age. Yes, it does take a lot of work to keep our bodies healthy and in a pain free state as you age. It is not God's desire for us to live in pain and suffering. 3 John 2: *Beloved, I pray that you may prosper in all things and be in health, just as your soul prospers.(NKJV).*

We can serve God and the body of Christ more effectively when we are in good health. Have you prayed for direction regarding your health? Are you an active participant or are you passive regarding your health?

At any age, if you do not take care of your health and well being, eventually you will suffer, have pain and your body which is the temple of God (1 Cor. 6:19-20) , will deteriorate faster than normal. Parents can be role models for their children by exposing them to healthy lifestyle habits. This is critical at a time when the U.S. has an obesity health concern and children are getting adult diseases such as Type 2 diabetes.

According to Dr. David Katz of the Yale Prevention Research Center, "this will be the first generation of children not to outlive their parents." One in three children born in the year 2000 is predicted to develop diabetes and...by the age of 12, 70% will have some hardening of the arteries. This is happening now! What you eat and the lifestyle you are modeling will not only affect your health, it will affect the health of your descendants for years to come.

Recent research show, diseases are partly the result of how your genes interact with your behaviors, such as your diet, physical activity, and your environment. If you have a family health history of a disease, you are more likely to get that disease yourself, but you can take steps to prevent disease by implementing healthy lifestyle choices. We can make a positive difference in the health of our family line for current and future generations.

Chapter 5
Our Environment

The biblical catastrophic flood was universal which means global and covered the mountains for 150 days; Genesis *7-19-20 and 24: And the waters prevailed exceedingly upon the earth; and all the high hills, that were under the whole heaven, were covered. Fifteen cubits upward did the waters prevail; and the mountains were covered.....also* ²⁴*And the waters prevailed upon the earth an hundred and fifty days. (KJV)* It also caused extreme changes in the global environment.

One of the changes was the elimination of the thermal blanket which is similar to the firmament in (Genesis 1). The thermal blanket created the greenhouse effect which controlled the climate, promoted growth of vegetation and protected the earth from radiation.

There was also a change in the atmospheric pressure. In reading several definitions of *Atmospheric pressure*, also called *barometric pressure*, it is the weight of the atmosphere pushing down on itself and the surface below which includes the sea. Merriam Webster defines Atmospheric pressure as: the pressure exerted in every direction at any given point by the weight of the atmosphere. National Geographic describes Atmospheric pressure as: The air around you has weight, and it presses against everything it touches. It is also called air pressure. It is the force exerted on a surface by the air above it as gravity pulls it to Earth.

We now know that higher atmospheric pressure can kill diseases and slow the aging process. There are several organizations developing equipment to simulate atmospheric pressure at a specific level to heal various diseases. For example, the Mayo Clinic now provide hyperbaric oxygen therapy which involves breathing pure oxygen in a pressurized room or tube. This is a well-established treatment for decompression sickness and is also used for serious infections, bubbles of air in your blood vessels, and wounds that won't heal as a result of diabetes or radiation injury. The Richmond Hyperbaric Health Clinic located in Canada treat patients for anti-aging and health management of childhood epilepsy and autism, cerebral palsy and diabetes-neuropathy.

According to Dr. Charles "Chuck" Missler, who is an Evangelical Christian, founder of Koinonia House, Bible teacher and author, with a physics background, it is believed the atmospheric pressure was 2:1 prior to the flood and is the reason men lived to 900 years and beyond, prior to the flood. After the flood, the atmospheric pressure ratio was reduced to an estimated ratio of 1:1. According to National Geographic and other sources, the current atmospheric differs based on your geographical location.

We have very little control over our environment today. The EPA is a Government agency, that monitors the quality of air, water, chemical, toxins, the effects of common pollutants on our health and etc. Depending on where you live the quality of air may contain pollutants such as, lead, ground level ozone, nitrogen dioxide (burning fuel from vehicles), sulfur oxides (emissions from power and industrial plants), and mold air spores.

The Huffington Post and Environmental Working Group (EWG) both published findings from a Body Burden which is a test that analyzes the chemicals in our blood. According to the results the average person has 91 toxic chemicals in their bodies, most of which did not exist 75 years ago. Several of the chemicals found in their blood are linked to serious health problems. What can we control?

Nutrition - *what we eat, drink and how often*. A good balanced diet is key. The USDA currently recommend 5-9 servings of fruits and vegetables a day.

I am excited about this study published in 2017! Research scientists from Imperial College London wanted to investigate how much fruit and vegetables you need to eat to gain the maximum protection against disease, and premature death," Dr. Dagfinn Aune, lead author of the research from the School of Public Health at Imperial College London, said "Our results suggest that although five portions of fruit and vegetables is good, ten a day is even better."

The results showed that even smaller amounts of fruits and vegetables have some protective benefits. For example, consuming 200 grams of fruits and vegetables per day – equivalent to two and a half servings – was associated with a 4 percent reduction in risk of cancer, and a 15 percent reduction in the risk of premature death.

Eating 10 portions of fruits and vegetables per day was tied to a:

- 24 percent reduced risk of heart disease.

- 33 percent reduced risk of stroke.

- 28 percent reduced risk of cardiovascular disease.

- 13 percent reduced risk of cancer.

- 31 percent reduction in premature death.

The research team took into account various factors such as a person's weight, smoking habits, physical activity levels, and overall diet, but the benefits of fruits and vegetables remained.

In 2015 the CDC estimated only 1 and 10, adults ate enough fruits and vegetables which is a combination of 5 cups.

Are you aware that major but unnoticeable changes start taking place in your body while in your 30s? In your 30s your brain starts to shrink, your hormones and muscle mass start to decrease, your taste buds start to change and more. It is a gradual change which you may not notice until you are in your 40s.

Fruits and vegetables provide essential vitamins and minerals, fiber, 1000s of phytonutrients and other substances that are important for good health, strengthening your immune system and longevity.

Water helps to lubricate and cushion joints, protects your spinal cord and sensitive tissues, get rid of wastes and keeps your body temperature normal. Initially you may find it challenging drinking one half your body weight in ounces or 8 glasses of water, however your body will later appreciate it.

As Dr William Sears would say, "go fishing"; eat fish such as salmon, tuna, halibut, and sardines 2 to 3 days a week, to improve brain and cardiovascular health.

There are electronic devices to help you track your meals. Exhibit C is a manual meal and exercise tracker to help you get started in monitoring what you currently eat and what changes you may want to consider.

Physical Activity - *how and when we move.* 66% of adults 65 years and over do have leisure time and exercise.* Regular physical activity is one of the most important things older adults can do for their health. Physical activities help the body to make its own medicine to fight disease, sleep better, improve mental health, strengthen bones, muscles and more.

According to the *2008 Physical Activity Guidelines for Americans*, older adults need to do two types of physical activities each week to improve health—aerobic and muscle-strengthening. For best results, adults 65 and older should exercise 150 minutes of moderate exercise or 75 minutes of vigorous exercise weekly.

According to *Harvard Health Publishing*, Stretching is just as important as exercise. Stretching keeps the muscles flexible, strong, and healthy. We need flexibility to maintain a range of motion in the joints. Without stretching, the muscles shorten and become tight. When you call on the muscles for activity, they are weak and unable to extend all the way. This puts you at risk for joint pain, strains, and muscle damage.

Exercise and stretching can also help you to relax and de-stress, which is important for longevity. There are electronic devices to help you track your physical activity. Exhibit C, is a meal and exercise tracker to help you get started in monitoring your exercise, movement activities and other changes you may want to consider.

Attitude and lifestyle -- 20% of adults 55 years and older suffer with mental distress associated with limitations in daily activities, physical impairments, grief following loss of loved ones, or challenging living arrangements, depression and substance abuse (CDC). Approximately 25% of adults aged 65 years and older have some type of mental health problem, such as a mood disorder not associated with normal aging (CDC).

Family and social support are important. Stay in a positive environment such as your church or social group. Develop healthy relationships with family and friends you can depend on. Keep negative people at a distance. Have open discussions with your doctor and ask questions.

My 89 years young mother is an excellent example of the importance of family support and taking control. About four years ago, my mother started having long periods of depression and fighting to maintain her independence. While preparing a care package for her, I included "Gems from Lady Mae", by Mae L. Blake, one of my mother's favorite people. I totally forgot about the book. One day, my mother called with excitement, expressing how much she enjoyed the book. My mother said, "after reading the book, I asked why am I sitting around feeling sorry for myself?"

Instead of sitting in the house feeling sorry for herself, between my sisters in New York and Iowa, she started asking them to schedule access-a-ride trips to the mall, in order to get out the house. During her trips she reads the newspaper and has breakfast. She also has my sisters make airline reservations to travel to various cities visiting family members and attending conferences. Local and long distance travelling is a big challenge for my mother because she is hearing impaired. My mother will tell you it is not easy; and she believes in prayer. It does not matter if your children or family members are near or far, they can still provide support in some way.

Making one positive change can have a domino effect. My mother has a one-story flight of stairs to climb. She shared some days, she wanted to leave the house, but the thought of going down and up the stairs was a discouragement. The stairs are not only a challenge for her, my sisters, brother and I no longer run up and down the stairs like we use to. My mother started 2017 off by investing in a chairlift. Now, the stairs are no longer a challenge for her.

Develop a plan to eliminate challenges, that are keeping you from achieving your goals. First, do not focus on limitations, instead focus on your goals, dreams and desires and second, put them in order of priority. Third, list the resources, people, and connections, available to you in accomplishing the first item on your list; in the order of what is easy to implement first and work your way through the list until the first goal is accomplish. All things are possible with God.

Sleep -- Wakefield Medical Inc did a recent sleep study. After doing some research, I now have a lot of respect for sleep. The amount of sleep you get is instrumental in quality of life issues. However, 49% of Americans are not getting enough sleep. A NIH, 2017, publication "Brain Basic: Understanding Sleep", shows 5 stages of sleep. Our brain is active and our body actually produces a hormone melatonin which is good for brain health such as Alzheimer's prevention and relieving stress. Lack of sleep can put into motion serious health challenges such as gut health, stress, weight gain, memory loss, cognitive function and etc are linked to lack of sleep. Adequate sleep, which is around 7-8 hours for adults, will help to improve your overall health, mental attitude, improved memory, and etc

Pills and Skills Model - Dr. William Sears makes reference to pills and skills model. Instead of asking your doctor what can I take, ask your doctor what can I do. This will alert your doctor that you want to be responsible for your health. Instead of your doctor thinking what can I prescribe, your doctor will think, what can I advise. Knowing your health numbers is important. You can write your numbers in Exhibit B. Be an active participant in your healthcare by reviewing your annual physical or test results, compare results to previous years, have a "pills and skills" discussion with your doctor in order to develop a plan of action to take your health to the next level. There is always room for improvement.

Chapter 6
Living Longer

People are living longer now; however, their bodies are in poor conditions; yes, pain and suffering. In a Gallup poll published in May 2014, 49% of retirees said they left the workforce earlier than they planned because of health problems or disability. The US Government goal for 2020 and now 2030 is to improve health, function and quality of life for older adults.

According to the CDC, chronic conditions such as heart disease, high blood pressure, cancer, and diabetes were the leading causes of death among U.S. adults age 65 and older in 2007–2009. People with more than one chronic conditions have a diminished quality of life and loss of independence. They have long periods of decline and disability. As functional ability—physical, mental, or both—further decline, people may lose the ability to perform more basic activities, called activities of daily living, such as taking care of themselves.

Health challenges, in terms of various disease and illness, have changed over the years; leprosy, tuberculosis, various plaques, and malaria are still around and we are now able to treat these diseases. We now have new challenges such as HIV/AIDs, various cancers, heart disease, influenza and etc. As previously mentioned, *today we have children with adult illnesses such as type 2 diabetes and are obese.*

Polo One publishes scientific research papers. One of the papers was Death and Oldest Old: Attitudes and

---

Preferences for End-of-Life-Care. They surveyed 42 oldest olds; oldest old are ages 95 to 101. Most felt ready to die, describing "waiting for it to happen", crying because they are still here. Others felt they should have died in their 80s. Instead of talking about dying, they were wondering why are they still here. Some oldest old, still have a will to live, remained strong...Yay!!

Churches can play an active role in keeping their members, who are seniors and oldest old actively involved and engaged in living life:

(1) Include them in a regular home visitation program or follow-up call list.

(2) Provide convenient options for them to get to church (the purpose of convenient is to reduce stress and make the seniors feel valued)

(3) Assist them in getting the necessary government assistance and services or making them aware of government services through workshops, newsletters, mailings, and etc.

(4) Senior Health Fairs to include health screening, consultation and referral for assistance.

(5) Social support events such as luncheons, movies, travel and etc, along with activities that pair them up with younger generations similar to mentoring.

(6) Promote physical activities such as walking, exercise, stretching, and etc

(7) Workshops on health and nutrition, electronic technology, motivational, movement, finance, scam awareness, safety, goal setting, ministry and etc

As a vendor, at a health fair in 2017, I had the pleasure of talking to a wonderful " older old" senior. I kept in touch with her and she celebrated her 100th birthday May 7, 2018. She shared that according to her doctor, she is in good health. She does not need a walker, wheelchair or cane, she still drives herself and others to appointments and shopping. She said she eats healthy and does floor exercises every morning. She said people often ask her how does she get up from the floor?...LOL. She is a retired nurse, and is surprised about the poor health of the young people today. She said, "I try to talk to younger people but they don't want to hear what I have to say". She started talking about her family members who have died, and said "I do wonder why I am still here". I said "you have a purpose, you are here because you are helping others." She said," you are right, each day I ask God who can I help today"?

VOICE LIFE

Chapter 7
Golden Advice

Super-centenarian: Super-centenarian is someone who lived to or past 110 years of age with documentation of the birth. The current longest living person in modern day is Jeanne Louise Calment.

In modern day history, Jeanne Louise Calment is one of my favorite super-centenarians and the oldest documented person who lived to be 122 years, 164 days old. Ms. Calment lived in France, she was born February 21, 1875 and died August 4ᵗʰ 1997. Researchers said her longevity was due to no stress because she never worked. Ms. Calment once said, "If you can't do anything about it, don't worry about it." She was very active, she played tennis, rode a bicycle, went swimming, roller skating, played the piano and enjoyed the opera. On her 100th birthday, she rode a bicycle around town thanking everyone for celebrating with her on her birthday. Ms. Calment shared her secret to longevity: she laughed a lot throughout her life, eating almost two pounds of chocolate a week, and frequently smeared olive oil on her skin.

As of April 2017 the oldest living super-centenarians is Ms. Violet Brown, who lives in Jamaica. She is 117 years and 136 days old. Worldwide it is estimated there are 150 to 600 super-centenarians; however, for various reason, it is difficult to verify all the ages. The USA has 27 super-centenarians. As of July 23, 2017, Ms. Delphine Gibson is the oldest living super-centenarians in the USA and she is 113 years and 176 days old. Ms.

Ida Joan is the second oldest also 113. Both have birthdays in August.

I first viewed Ms. Violet Brown's story on *Inside Edition.* At 117 years old, there is documentation showing Ms. Brown as the oldest living person. She has two caretakers and the help of her 97-year-old son who lives with her. Ms. Brown enjoys each and every day and walks short distances with a cane. She is crediting hard work as a cane farmer, and her Catholic faith to her long life along with her diet. Ms. Brown said, she doesn't eat chicken or pork but will dine on just about anything else. *YouTube* video (April 2017): *InsideEdition.com - Keleigh Nealon*

There are several *YouTube videos of Mr. Richard Arvin Overton.* He was born May 11, 1906 and is the oldest living World War II veteran. He turned 111 years old in May of 2017. Mr. Overton shared, he was still driving on a video posted when he was 109. In a YouTube video posted in May 2017 and another July 2017, Mr. Overton said, he can still walk, hear and see; and he has no pain or aches. He loves the celebrity status he is receiving. Mr. Overton met and had breakfast with President Obama, at the White House. He enjoys smoking cigars (he made it clear, he does not inhale) and he put one teaspoon of whiskey in his coffee. Mr. Overton said he does not know how much longer he will live, but every day he lives he has more fun.

Centenarian is someone who lives to and or beyond 100 years of age. According to the 2010 Census the USA has 53,364 centenarians. A CNN article, *Living to 100, The*

Centenarian Tide is on the Rise, January 25, 2016, the USA had 72,197 centenarians.

A YouTube video of Jessie P. Jordon was produced by Denise Lodde and published 2010. Ms. Jessie Jordon was asked, what is it like being 105? She said, it is interesting, you never know when your next minute is. Ms. Jordon enjoyed swimming, stayed active all her life and stopped swimming at age 101. Her secret to longevity and happiness is peace from knowing God and forgiveness. Ms. Jordon said she is ready for heaven, I had to laugh when she said "I nearly made it there a couple of times and was disturbed. It was not nice coming back"…LOL   Jessie Jordon finally made it to heaven February 12, 2011.

I did not have an opportunity to interview any of the centenarians nor the super-centenarian, but I really enjoyed viewing their YouTube video and reading the various articles about them. There are several inspirational *YouTube* videos spotlighting centenarians and allowing them to share their story. If you know any one beyond 3 score and 10 take the time to listen to them.

VOICE LIFE

Chapter 8
Inspiring Others and Ourselves

As we inspire our young people to achieve their dreams and goals, we need to inspire our older generation to do the same. There is something for us to do at each stage of our life. Now that your children are grown, your grandchildren are grown, and maybe the great-grand-children are grown, you have more free time, why not work on your dreams? The late Dr. Myles Munroe shared on several occasions the wealthiest place on earth is the cemetery because you have books that were never written, a painting that was never painted, music never written, poetry never read, businesses never open. You are never too young or old to focus on a healthier lifestyle in order to accomplish your dream.

Mrs. Betty Soskin is currently in her 90s and working in 2017. I enjoy reading articles and watching her YouTube videos. I first heard about Mrs. Soskin several years ago while watching the news and became a fan. In watching several YouTube videos of Mrs. Soskin, I found out she became a Park Ranger at age 85. She is now 96 years old and the oldest Park Ranger with the National Park Service in Richmond, Ca. In the *YouTube video "Ties That Bind"* Mrs. Soskin shared that she is proud to have made it to, at that time, age 93. She shared that not all her years were proud years. Her survival depended on being able to relate to others and keep herself whole enough. She stated no one can survive this world alone. Mrs. Soskin is still actively working. She was born September 22, 1921.

I would like to share the stories of Mr.Horace Sheffield and Ms. Amy Craton who both returned to college and graduated in 2017:

Mr. Horace Sheffield of Barnesville, Georgia, completed a lifelong goal to graduate college in May of 2017, at the age of 88. Mr. Sheffield dropped out of college in 1965 to help educate his daughter. According to the ABC news article, he said:

"I'm retired and living on fixed income, and I did not think I could go to college and pay tuition," said Sheffield. "But when I saw this article that senior citizens could go to college for free, Shorter accepted me at no tuition. I paid a $200 graduation fee and that's all I paid. I walked with a walker."

Ms. Amy Craton received her degree in January 2017 at the age of 94 from Southern New Hampshire University with a GPA of 4.0. Ms Craton had put her education on hold in 1962 to return to work and raise her four children following a divorce.

Although I mentioned Mr. Sheffield and Ms Craton there are lots of stories of seniors returning to school to complete their education goals or obtaining degrees.

Zeb McDowell, "my uncle", is amazing. He was inducted into the Mt Holly Sports Hall of Fame in August 2015. At the time he was 83. In 1953 he graduated from Reid High in Belmont. He received college scholarship offers from schools such as North Carolina A&T. Due to the death of my grandfather, my uncle instead chose to stay home and help his family. At age 55, he retired from Duke Energy after 36 years on the job and started his own construction company. At 85 he is still actively involved in his construction company handling major contracts, at the church where he is as a deacon and trustee, and at home as a husband who loves to cook and bake.

Mother Workman, is a woman of faith who believes in prayer and consecration. She was the founder of Christian Haitian Outreach (CHO). In February of 1994, I was invited to travel to Haiti on a mission trip, with West Angeles COGIC World Missions Department as part of the Skid Row Ministry team. I had the pleasure of meeting Mother Eleanor Workman. As we toured the grounds, I was inspired and blessed to see what Mother Workman was able to accomplish with the help of God in Haiti such as the orphanage and dormitories. I enjoyed listening to the children sing. In a January 2000 Charisma Magazine article "No Such Thing As Retirement", Mother Workman at the age of 80 years old stated she doesn't have any plans of slowing down. In 2009, on YouTube, Mother Workman shared CHO's latest project at that time was the completion of a beautiful clinic for Jesus. She was almost 90 and still going strong. Mother Workman went to her heavenly home in May of 2017.

Track and Field – Do you want a second chance for a track and field metal? USA Track and Field (USATF) has a category for ages 95-99 and 100 plus.

Julia "Hurricane" Hawkins and Idea Keeling Ms. Keeling is the first women to complete in the 100 meters at the age 100 years old. She is the 60 meter world record holder for 95-99 age group. She was the world record holder for the 60 meters with a time of 58.34 for the 100 plus age group until March of 2018 when Ms. Hawkins broke the record of 24.79 seconds. *Orville Rogers* is the current record holder of the men's 60 meters with a record of 19.13 seconds, for the 100 plus age group.

If you want another chance for a track and field metal, start getting in shape now. For additional information regarding sign ups, Google USATF Masters Indoors Championships or RunnerSpace.

Chapter 9
Abundant Life

John 10:10 - *The thief cometh not, but for to steal, and to kill, and to destroy: I am come that they might have life, and that they might have it more abundantly.(KJV)*

I like the King James version because it talks about life more abundantly which is described as the fullness of joy and strength for mind, body, and soul. Today "being in health" is not described as the absence of disease, disability, or illness; it is well-being. Well-being takes into account the total person; mind, body and soul to include physical, economic, social, emotional, and psychological well-being. Increased risk factors which lower your well-being such as unhealthy eating habits, sedentary lifestyle, lack of sleep, chronic stress, illness, disease and etc without preventive action, can lead to premature death. Higher well-being is associated with decreased risk of illness and injury, improved immune system, prayer and meditation, social relationships, education and positive activities leading to increased longevity. (See Figure 2 – next page) What are you doing to move towards a Higher Well-Being?

Prime-Time Health, written by Dr. William Sears, MD, has a section on the Secrets of Centenarians and list the following longevity-boosting habits that help them to reach 100 years old:

THE ILLNESS / WELLNESS CONTINUUM

WELLNESS PARADIGM

PRE-MATURE DEATH | Disability Symptoms Signs | Awareness Education Growth | HIGH-LEVEL WELLNESS

TREATMENT PARADIGM

© 1972, 1975, 1981, 1988,
NEUTRAL POINT
(NO DISCERNABLE ILLNESS OR WELLNESS)

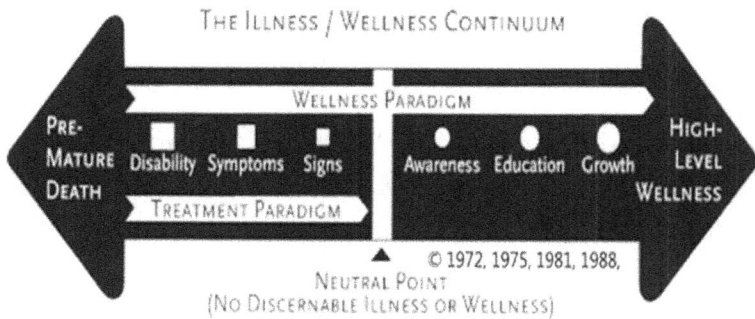

Figure 2: Jack Travis' Illness-Wellness Continuum

Move -   Active centenarians spend much of their day doing physical exercise, such as gardening, walking or on a golf course. Your joints do not have a chance to get stiff and moving helps the body to make its own medicine.

Love - They have deep intimate relationships.

They're lean – As they got older, they neither gained fat nor lost muscle.

They eat less – Centenarians generally eat 10 to 20% fewer daily calories than people on the standard American diet.

They graze – they eat smaller meals several times a day and they take their time eating.

They eat pure – they eat real foods, mainly fruits, vegetables and fish.

They laugh and have fun – They enjoy themselves, fun activities and humor is good therapy.

They pray – Spiritual beliefs and practice occupy most of their time and thoughts. It gives them a sense of spiritual belonging.

They're flexible - The most adaptable live the longest.

They serve – Volunteering and ministering to others.
They're musical – Music mellows the mind.
They swim – Water is a refuge, calming the mind and relaxing the body.
They think – Mental exercise, crosswords puzzles, keeps their mind active.
They sleep – Quality sleep is very important.
They're up!! – They are positive thinkers and they do not worry about anything they cannot change.
They work – They need a project, a reason to wake up in the morning.
They're sexy – Couples who engage in sexual activity tend to live the longest.
They plan – Set goals for the next 5 to 10 years.

Voice life! Abide in the word of God. Proverbs 18:21 *Death and life are in the power of the tongue: and they that love it shall eat the fruit thereof.(KJV)*.

One of my favorite scriptures is Philippians 4:8 *Finally, brethren, whatsoever things are true, whatsoever things are honest, whatsoever things are just, whatsoever things are pure, whatsoever things are lovely, whatsoever things are of good report; if there be any virtue, and if there be any praise, think on these things. (KJV)*

Proverbs 17:22 *A merry heart doeth good like a medicine: but a broken spirit drieth the bones. (KJV)*

Exhibit A has an abundant life assessment.

VOICE LIFE

Chapter 10
My Grandma Rose

Grandma Rose was born December 19, 1906 and died September 24, 2007. She was 100 and 287 days old. Grandma Rose and her two brothers were close. She was the oldest, and they often visited each other and talked on the phone. I regret not making it to more family reunions and taking pictures because now all I have is a memory of my grandmother and her two brothers sitting together at the table as we greeted them with smiles, hugs and kisses.

Grandma Rose's brothers both died within weeks of each other and she wanted to join them. At the time, she was in her late 70s. She said her children were grown, and she was no longer needed. My family's mission was to let her know she was needed. My mother encouraged us to start calling her on a regular basis and Grandma Rose recovered from her state of depression. Several years later she ended up saving her youngest daughter's life and we were quick to remind her that God has a plan for her life. Because she decided to live, her daughter now lives. It is important to have ongoing communication with our seniors and older old, to let them know they are needed, show them love and encouragement.

 A few years before Grandma Rose's 100ᵗʰ birthday, we noticed she was always dusting, sweeping the floor and cleaning the house. I said grandma, why are you constantly cleaning. She said, "they came for me but they said I was not ready. They said my house was not clean". Grandma Rose was unable to tell me who said her house was not clean. She was cleaning like it was physical; however I felt it was spiritual.

Grandma Rose had a beautiful 100 birthday party and she refused to walk with a cane. My Uncle escorted her into their church dining area where she was greeted by family and friends. About three months prior to Grandma Rose's 101 birthday, she basically stopped eating and she joined her brothers in heaven several weeks after. Her house was finally clean.

Now we are inspiring my mother who is 89 and her three surviving siblings. My mother was diagnosed with thyroid cancer when she was about 26 years old. She was raising 5 children. She said at the time, she asked God to let her live to see her children grown; that was her purpose. God blessed her with life, another husband, two more children and to see her grandchildren and great-grandchildren to mature into adults.

Chapter 11
Are You Living Out God's Purpose For Your Life or Are You Taking A Short Cut?

As a teenager, my mother would tell me, I was not going to live to see my 21st birthday. Although I pretended to ignored her, subconsciously I believed her. Turning 18, which was the legal age in New York at the time, was no big deal for me. However, once I realized I was months away from turning 21 years old, there were feelings of excitement and mixed concerns about making it. A countdown started within me. The day I turned 21, I called my mother and said, "I made it!" Neither my mother nor I realized the mental impact it made on me. I remember a feeling of release and a feeling of joy when the day finally arrived.

Be thankful to God, show love, understanding and forgiveness each day. Death can happen at any age. It does not discriminate and there are all types of statistical information available to prove it. When you know you are in right standing with God, you can enjoy life. So, I ask the question, **are you living out God's purpose for your life?**

 Although Moses was raised by Pharaoh's daughter with special privileges when compared to his brethrens, and familiar with their culture, he knew in his heart, he was not an Egyptian. At the age of 40, he went out looking for answers. For us this might be searching Google, Ancestry.com, FamilyTree.com, Facebook and in the Library. In Moses search for answers, he killed an

Egyptian and had to flee Egypt.

Moses starts a new life in the land of Midian. He was contented living with his wife, grown children, his extended family and taking care of sheep and goats when God called him at 80 years of age to lead the Israelites out of Egypt. Moses was probably thinking why me? I am too old, I just want to relax, I have moved on. He was not expecting God to call him at 80, however, with age comes wisdom. Research published in the *Psychological Science Publication,* concluded that older people are better decision makers when the rewards are tied to outcome.

Although God prepared Moses for the assignment, he lacked confidence in his ability to accomplish it. Exodus 3:11 (NKJV) But Moses said to God, "Who am I that I should go to Pharaoh, and that I should bring the children of Israel out of Egypt?" However, God said, I will certainly be with you. When God gives you an assignment, he will:

- anoint you,

- equip you, and

- empower you.

You do not have to leave your home to answer God's call. Initially Moses did not feel confident, yet a powerful prayer warrior was within him. His intercessory prayers gave the Israelites something to focus on besides pain and suffering. In Psalm 90:12-17, Moses is asking God to have mercy and compassion on his people.

He asked God to help them to grow in understanding and wisdom, Job 12:12 - *Is not wisdom found among the aged? Does not long life bring understanding? James 1:5 - If any of you lacks wisdom, let him ask God, who gives generously to all without reproach, and it will be given him. (NIV)*

Ask God to reveal his glory not only to us but also our children. I have asked God on several occasions to reveal himself to my daughter in a special way to increase her faith and knowledge of his greatness. I have shared my experience with her, but there is nothing like having your own experience. I know Moses' mother prayed over him as she nursed him. What mother would pass up that opportunity?

 2 Corinthian 4:6 – For God, who commanded the light to shine out of darkness, hath shined in our hearts, to give the light of the knowledge of the glory of God in the face of Jesus Christ. (KJV)

Moses was 120 years old when he died and in good health. According to Deuteronomy 34:7, Moses lost neither his eyesight nor his strength before and was not diminished in body or mind by old age. Moses stayed actively involved, he was living life, he was an intercessor, he was not living day by day waiting for death.

Aaron accepted God's call to be Moses' spokesman at the age of 83. He and Moses had a close relationship. He was the first High Priest of Israelites, married with children. Aaron was 123 years old when he died. The

Bible did not mention any deteriorating health. (Numbers 33:39).

God told both Moses and Aaron when their transition period was near and their successor. God is still speaking to us today.

Galatians 6:9-10 – *And let us not be weary in well doing: for in due season we shall reap, if we faint not. As we have therefore opportunity, let us do good unto all men, especially unto them who are of the household of faith. (KJV)*

❖

Roman 10:9-10 - *If you declare with your mouth, "Jesus is Lord," and believe in your heart that God raised him from the dead, you will be saved. For it is with your heart that you believe and are justified, and it is with your mouth that you profess your faith and are saved. (NIV)*

VOICE LIFE

EXHIBIT A

Abundant Life Assessment

Considering you are now going to live beyond 3 score and 10 what can you do to make your life more abundant? What about travelling, finishing school or obtaining a degree, new hobby, new ministry, new career, new friends, sports activity or etc.

1.   What steps can you take to accomplish it?

    (a)   What is your time frame?

    (b)   How will you feel after you accomplish it?

2.   What gift/talents are you blessed with?

3.   How are you currently using your gift/talents?

4.   What steps can you take to improve your health?

**This self-assessment is just a start,
write the vision and make it plain. Habakkuk 2:2.**

EXHIBIT B

Know your numbers

A1c Blood Glucose _____   **Date**_____

Cholesterol

LDL____

HDL_____

Total Cholesterol _____   **Date**_____

Triglyceride_____   **Date**_____

Blood Pressure _____ / _____

PSA Level _____

Waist _____

Weight _____

Favorite Bible Scripture(s):

_____

_____

EXHIBIT C-1

Meal and Exercise Tracker

Week____ Date ____	Your Goals	Day 1	Day 2	Day 3	Day 4	Day 5	Day 6	Day 7
Real Food Portions								
Vegetables - variety # of Servings								
Fruits/Berries – variety # of Servings								
Breakfast Did you have breakfast?								
Water- # of ounces								
Exercises-How many minutes								
W=Walking; **R**=Running; **C**=Cycling; **P**=Push-up; **S**=Set-Ups; **St**=Stretch **Wts**=Weights								
Sleep –How many hours								
Social Events/Church								
Junk Food-sweets, chips, and etc								
Other:								
Other:								

EXHIBIT C-2

Meal and Exercise Tracker

Week____ Date ____	Your Goals	Day 1	Day 2	Day 3	Day 4	Day 5	Day 6	Day 7
Real Food Portions								
Vegetables - variety # of Servings								
Fruits/Berries – variety # of Servings								
Breakfast Did you have breakfast?								
Water- # of ounces								
Exercises-How many minutes								
W=Walking; **R**=Running; **C**=Cycling; **P**=Push-ups; **S**=Set-Ups; **St**=Stretch **Wts**=Weights								
Sleep –How many hours								
Social Events/Church								
Junk Food-sweets, chips, and etc								
Other:								
Other:								

References

Books:

- Spirit Filled Life Bible – Church of God In Christ
- Matthew Henry's Commentary on the Whole Bible, 1996
- The New Strong's Exhaustive Concordance of The Bible, 1990
- Prime-Time Health, Authors: William Sears, MC with Martha Sears, RN (Oct 2010)
- Gems From Lady Mae, Author: Mae L. Blake

News:

ABC -Mr. Horace Sheffield http://abcnews.go.com/Lifestyle/88-year-georgia-man-graduates-college-wanted-degree/story?id=47272888

CBS - For a longer life, researchers say eat this many fruits and veggies per day https://www.cbsnews.com/news/for-a-longer-life-researchers-say-eat-this-many-fruits-and-veggies-per-day/

ESPN - 102-year-old's ace leads to spot on 'Tonight Show' http://www.espn.com/golf/news/story?id=2829770

NBC - Here's How Sleep Loss Can Affect Alzheimer's https://www.nbcnews.com/health/health-news/here-s-how-sleep-loss-can-affect-alzheimer-s-n781501

NBC Sports - http://olympics.nbcsports.com/2018/03/19/100-year-old-world-record-track-and-field-video/

Today -: Ms Amy Craton https://www.today.com/news/50-years-later-94-year-old-woman-graduates-college-4-t107141

USA Today - Parents who do the unthinkable -- kill their children - https://www.usatoday.com/story/news/nation/2014/09/10/parents-kill-children-fbi-data/15280259/

Los Angeles Times, Betty Reid Soskin: An assault on her is an assault on us all': U.S.' oldest park ranger beaten and robbed in her home, Los Angeles Times, by Veronica Rocha, July 2016 http://www.latimes.com/local/lanow/la-me-ln-oldest-park-ranger-robbed-beaten-20160630-snap-story.html

VOICE LIFE

Websites:

Addicted 2 Success - 10 Successful People Who Proved That Age is Nothing But A Number
https://addicted2success.com/news/10-succesful-people-who-proved-that-age-is-nothing-but-a-number/

Answer in Genesis – Longevity or Countdown
https://answersingenesis.org/contradictions-in-the-bible/longevity-or-countdown/

Bible Gateway https://www.biblegateway.com/

Brain Basics: Understanding Sleep
https://www.ninds.nih.gov/Disorders/Patient-Caregiver-Education/Understanding-Sleep

CDC – Depression
https://www.cdc.gov/mentalhealth/data_stats/depression.htm

CDC Genomics and disease
https://www.cdc.gov/genomics/disease/genomic_diseases.htm

CDC – Morbidity and Mortality Weekly Report - Adults Meeting Fruit and Vegetable Intake Recommendations — United States, 2013.
https://www.cdc.gov/mmwr/preview/mmwrhtml/mm6426a1.htm

CDC - Only 1 In 10 Adults Get Enough Fruits or Vegetables
https://www.cdc.gov/media/releases/2017/p1116-fruit-vegetable-consumption.html

CDC - Physical Activity
https://www.cdc.gov/healthyplaces/healthtopics/physactivity.htm
https://www.cdc.gov/media/releases/2017/p1116-fruit-vegetable-consumption.html

CDC – The State of Mental Health in Aging America
https://www.cdc.gov/aging/pdf/mental_health.pdf

Charisma Magazine   https://www.charismamag.com/site-archives/24-uncategorised/9416-theres-no-such-thing-as-retirement

CNN Living to 100
http://www.cnn.com/2016/01/25/health/centenarians-increase/index.html

Faith and Health Connections
http://www.faithandhealthconnection.org/5-reasons-why-god-wants-us-healthy-well-and-fit/

Harvard Health Publishing, Harvard Medical School: The Importance of Stretching: https://www.health.harvard.edu/staying-healthy/the-importance-of-stretching

International Journal of Epidemiology, Fruit and vegetable intake and the risk of cardiovascular disease, total cancer and all-cause mortality—a systematic review and dose-response meta-analysis of prospective studies https://academic.oup.com/ije/article/46/3/1029/3039477

Los Angeles Times, Betty Reid Soskin: An assault on her is an assault on us all': U.S.' oldest park ranger beaten and robbed in her home, Los Angeles Times, by Veronica Rocha, July 2016 http://www.latimes.com/local/lanow/la-me-ln-oldest-park-ranger-robbed-beaten-20160630-snap-story.html

Mayo Clinic - Hyperbaric oxygen therapy https://www.mayoclinic.org/tests-procedures/hyperbaric-oxygen-therapy/basics/definition/prc-20019167

Zeb McDowell, Gaston Gazette, by Richard Walker, 2015 Mount Holly Sports Hall of Fame: Four individuals and four teams to be inducted August 15, http://www.gastongazette.com/article/20150714/NEWS/150719519

Zeb McDowell, Mt. Holly Sports Hall of Fame to induct versatile athlete Zeb McDowell http://banner-news.com/mt-holly-sports-hall-of-fame-to-induct-versatile-athlete-zeb-mcdowell-p1762-94.htm   July 29, 2015

Dr. Charles "Chuck" Missler - Author, evangelical Christian, Bible teacher and The founder of the Koinonia House ministry in Idaho, Koinonia House Presents, An Expositional Commentary, the Book of Genesis, Session 11 Genesis 6.

NASA - Scientists Confirm Historic Massive Flood in Climate Change - https://www.nasa.gov/vision/earth/lookingatearth/abrupt_change.html

National Geographic: https://www.nationalgeographic.org/encyclopedia/atmospheric-pressure/

NCBI - Atmospheric pressure as a natural climate regulator for a terrestrial planet with a biosphere
https://www.ncbi.nlm.nih.gov/pmc/articles/PMC2701016/

NCBI - How old are you, really? Communicating chronic risk through 'effective age' of your body and organs
https://www.ncbi.nlm.nih.gov/pmc/articles/PMC4974726/
ww.ncbi.nlm.nih.gov/pubmed/20122036

NCBI - Place of death and end-of-life transitions experienced by very old people with differing cognitive status: retrospective analysis of a prospective population-based cohort aged 85 and over.
https://www.ncbi.nlm.nih.gov/pubmed/24317193

NCBI - The oldest old in the last year of life: population-based findings from Cambridge city over-75s cohort study participants aged 85 and older at death. https://www.ncbi.nlm.nih.gov/pubmed/20122036

NCBI - With age comes wisdom: decision making in younger and older adults.   https://www.ncbi.nlm.nih.gov/pubmed/21960248

PROS ONE - Death of the oldest old Attitudes and Preferences for End of Life-Care Qualitative Research within a Population-Based Cohort Study
 http://journals.plos.org/plosone/article?id=info:doi/10.1371/journal.pone.0150686

Psychological Science, 29 September 2011, With Age Comes Wisdom : Decision Making in Younger and Older Adults
https://pdfs.semanticscholar.org/705a/6a6b41b7d185410934b25fa291d5696d3280.pdf

Richmond Hyperbaric Health Center - Benefits of Hyperbaric Oxygen Therapy (HBOT) http://www.richmond-hyperbaric.com/benefits_of_hyperbaric_oxygen.html

Ashburn Sterling Internal Medicine and Pediatric, Author: Doreen Mattinmiro, MSN, FNP – You Are What You Eat:
 http://myhealthcare.org/news/you-are-what-you-eat

The Conversation – Health and Medicine
http://theconversation.com/heres-what-people-in-their-90s-really-think-about-death-58053

UC Davis Statistic – Oldest Women
http://anson.ucdavis.edu/~wang/calment.html

VOICE LIFE

UC San Diego Health: Aging Gracefully: 9 Things That Happen to Your Body (Some Aren't So Bad!
 https://health.ucsd.edu/news/features/Pages/2015-08-31-listicle-aging.aspx

YouTube Videos

- Viola Brown: Woman Credits Hard Work and Faith To Being New Oldest Living Person at 117, Inside Edition, Published April 18, 2017
- Jessie P. Jordon: 105 Year Old Lady Shares The Secret To Happiness, 100 Huntley, by Denise Lodde and Published Nov 3, 2010
- Mr. Richard Arvin Overton: 109-Year-Old Veteran and His Secrets to Life Will Make You Smile | Short Film Showcase, National Geographic, Published Feb 5, 2017
- Mr. Richard Arvin Overton: World's oldest WWII veteran turns 111, USA Today, Published May 12, 2017
- Mr. Richard Arvin Overton: Special Alpha Mission 111: Richard Overton, Cigar Dave Show, Published July 1, 2017
- Betty Reid Soskin: *Ties That Bind, SCC Public Health, Published, Feb 23, 2015*
- Betty Reid Soskin: Betty Reid Soskin's 95th bday celebrated, Mike Aldax, Published, Sept 24, 2016
- Eleanor Workman: *Mom Workman CHO Haiti July 2009,* ftccclayton, Published April 22, 2010.

VOICE LIFE

www.ingramcontent.com/pod-product-compliance
Lightning Source LLC
Chambersburg PA
CBHW070937280326
41934CB00009B/1912